PRACTICE SILENCE AND MEDITATION

SILENCE, MEDITATION, PEACE OF MIND AND STATE OF SAMADHI

JAYANTILAL SENDHABHAI PATEL

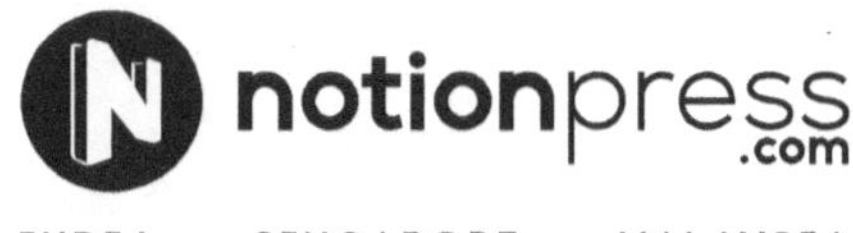

Notion Press

Old No. 38, New No. 6
McNichols Road, Chetpet
Chennai - 600 031

First Published by Notion Press 2020
Copyright © Jayantilal Sendhabhai Patel 2020
All Rights Reserved.

ISBN 978-1-64783-636-8

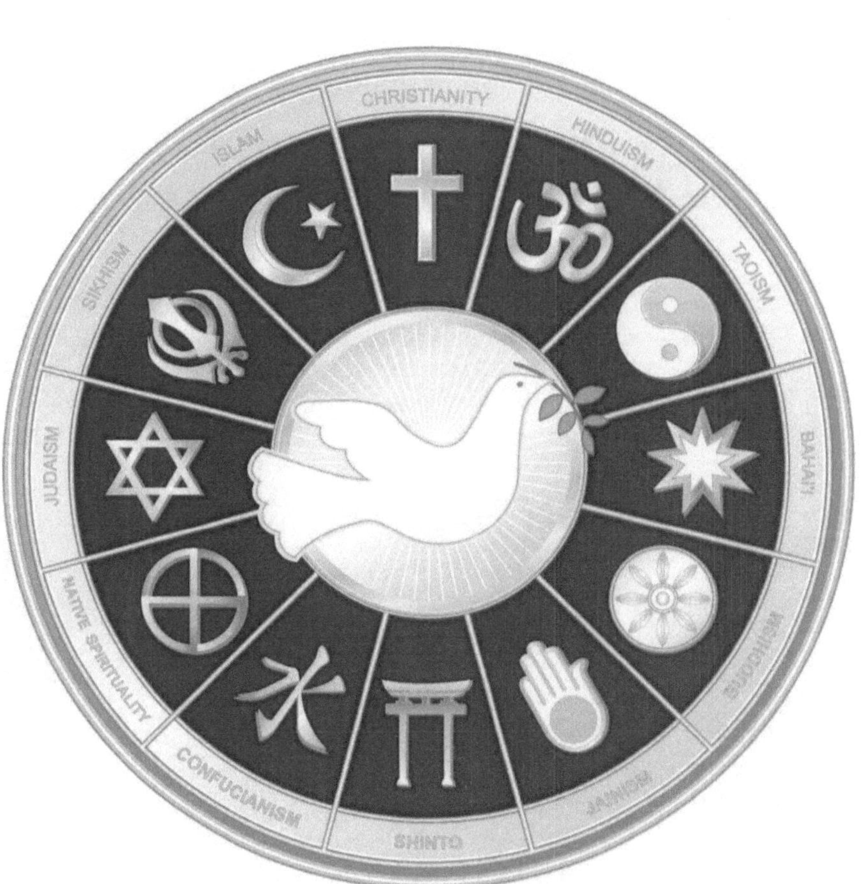

CHRISTIANITY
ISLAM
HINDUISM
SIKHISM
TAOISM
JUDAISM
BAHA'I
NATIVE SPIRITUALITY
BUDDHISM
CONFUCIANISM
JAINISM
SHINTO

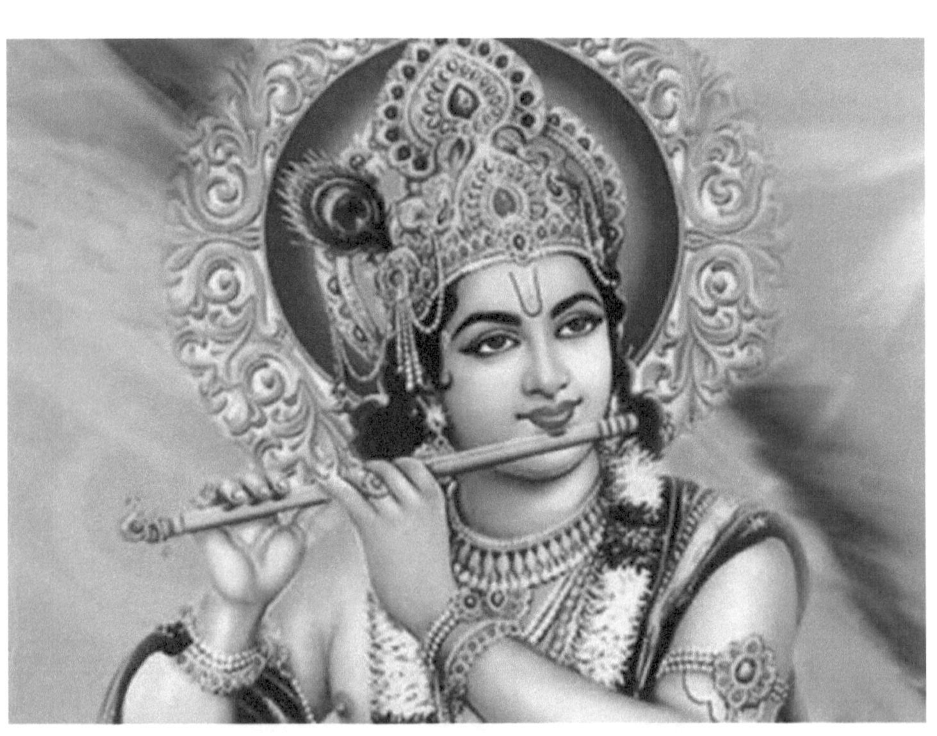

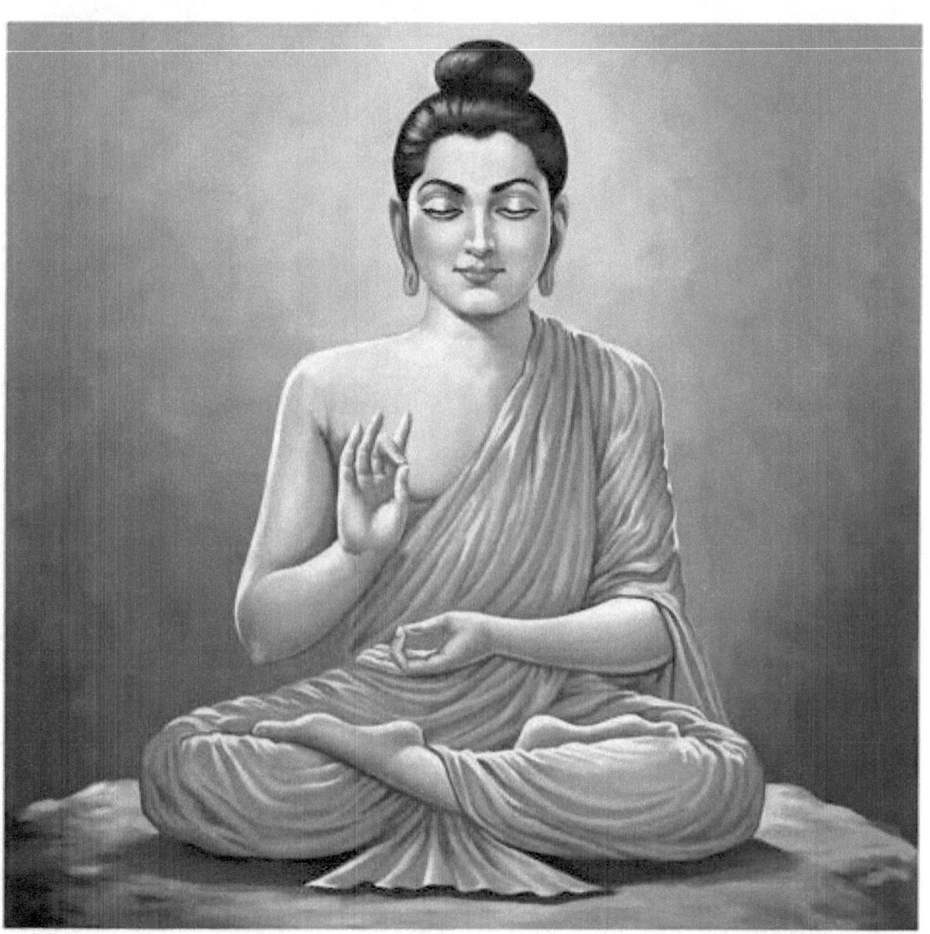

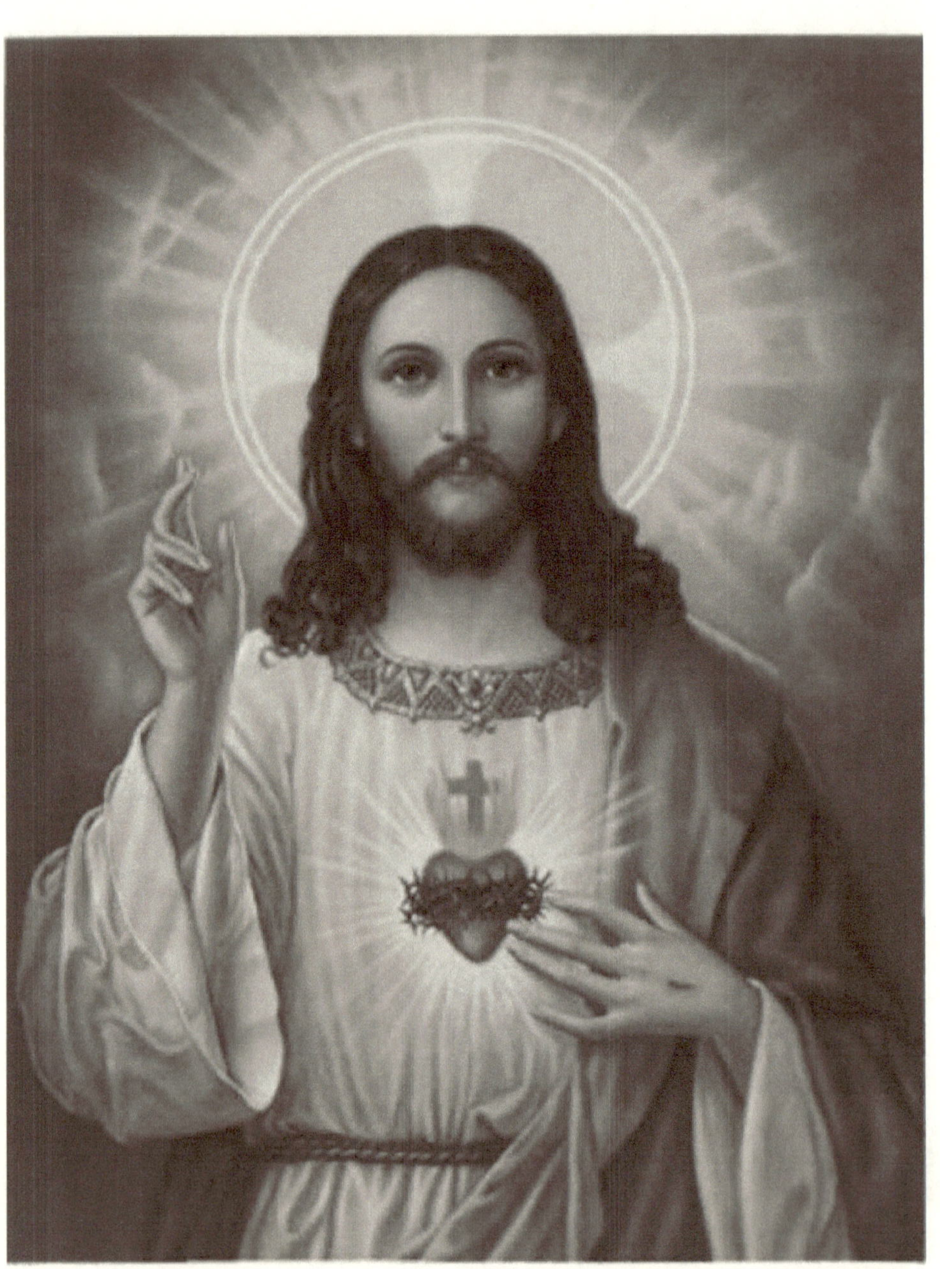

Readers can read my previous book

"Peace and Happiness"

The book contains philosophical thoughts for peace, harmony, love, happiness. There are guideline for being positive and come out from negative thoughts, how to come out depression and leave a peaceful life, importance of silence, save time, be humerous, impotant of forgiveness in life, how to understand others, how to increase internal energy, come out from criticizam, how to remain vigilant, how to maintain social relation, learn to give without back thoughts, be aware while carefree, cooperation to others, come out from anger, always focus on success of present moment, to be patience, to overcome difficulties, listen inner voice before action, be courageous for any situation, adopt calm posture in a situation of stress, pride leads to ridiculous battle, to be satisfied in present, be open minded, happiness has source in our mind, nothing without inconvience, maintain confidence, forget past and don't think for future, let live others happy for being happy, listen others, listen music in spare time to be calm etc.

Contents

Preface

I am Patel Jayantilal Sendhabhai, engineer and worked in projects at India and abroad. I have worked more than 60 nationalities persons and learned different cultures and customs from them. I have learned various meditation practices. I have written my book on "Practice Silence and Meditation" for people, who want peace, love and to be loved, happiness and work betterment of people, harmony and humanity. My effort of publishing this book will help them to live their life with peace and happiness. I thank all of you who helped me in this mission and request people to read and understand my book. You can contact me for any explanation and difficulties. Pardon me for my mistake and if anybody hurt by my attempt.

Thanks once again,

Ohm Tat Sat-Ohm Santir Bhavatu-Amen

Patel Jayantilal Sendhabhai
7824 Avenue Stuart, Montreal,
H3N 2R6, Quebec, Canada.
E-mail: pateljs2003@hotmail.com

Silence and Peace

Silence brings peace to someone. Mahatma Gandhi remains silent for some time in a day or week and advised person to remain two hours silent in a day. Buddha also advised to follow silence throughout the meditation session of about 7 week in past and now a day conducted one day to 45 days. Indian yogis also advised to practice silence to improve mediation quality and to get inner peace.

In general meaning it is understood by people that not to speak is silence. This is good but religious or meditation preacher advised to enlarge boundaries of silence. Person should keep away mobile, avoid listening radio or television. They should not read books or news papers or any literatures, they should not to look others face to face. They should try to be silent and avoid unnecessary thoughts coming to mind by daily activities. Some preacher's advice not to brush teeth, save and even not to seat for meditation just remains with nature. Mahatma Gandhi was give written instruction as and when required but it's not allowed to meditation practiosner.

When you are not speaking or trying for silence your inner silence or inner peace increases and you are entering in place of go to meditation. Silence avoids unnecessary arguments and dispute among friends, relative or coworkers and helps to enter inner peace. Small comments invites big war some time so silence or keep quiet resolve some issues.

Practicing silence or minimize activities reduce internal energy usage and hence loss. Normally person is not doing meditation his internal energy voltage may be 1.5 volts and person who reached very high level in meditation may have 16 volt energy potential so by keeping silence it start accumulating energy level in human body and increase quality of meditation hence inner peace.

You can say silence is directly affecting meditation level. Person keep more silence will have better and better meditation so all wise people or meditation practiosner like to remain calm or in silence. It reduces blood pressure level and stress level also and all deices or pain by improve internal flow in body organs will be discussed in later chapter.

One of police officer arranged meditation program in India to improve mental condition and stress on prisoners and found in their medical checkup the stress level was improved. In some government offices in India allow to attend 10 days meditation sessions and their leaves approved without deducting from their leave balance. The work performance due to silence and meditation improve. In some state it is compulsory to attend this course during their civil services training program.

When someone talks or speaks too much their mind become fickle and not allow them to do meditation. During silence stop speaking, giving sign or hints, giving writing instructions or direct face to face contact which stops mind fickleness comes down and meditation become stronger and better.

Person seeing things in outer world he gets thoughts out of which 70-80% negative ones and small one positive. If he goes to wise person or his preacher his mind becomes calm. Buddha suggested looking inward called "Vipassana" and following silence practice to make mind calm. When mind become calm bliss from universe enter to his body which flows to whole body is cleaning,deleting good or bad thoughts of previous and present incarnations which stored in unconscious mind. Religious preacher defined it as "Karmas or Shankaras".

While practicing silence outer sound should be minimum possible but in social life it's not possible so mediator preferred to go forest or lonely area. Preacher advice meditation practiosner to keep not to participate in outer noise, becoming witness and keep mind on breathe pattern or sound come out while breathing and change that to good meaningful words. These makes meditation better and mind peaceful and calm.

I read one incident described in book which I like to put here. One person came to attend meditation program in India from foreign country. He started his practice to remain silence and do meditation. He was not able to perform activities told him to do avec peace of mind, he thought or heard because centre was closed to vegetables and fish market form where too much sound was coming and he was getting disturbed. He gone to his preacher and told what he experienced. The preachers explained him to continue the practice, not to involve in outer noise and to outer world say to be witness, look into inner side and do the meditation. He followed instructions and completed 10 days meditation and experienced silence and peace of mind. He was very happy after the course. He accepted that fickleness of mind can be reduced and disturbance of outer world noise also avoided by this meditation practice.

I also faced same thing which I will describe here. Once I was attending 10 days silence and meditation program. I was having too much pain in legs as I was sitting about 10 hours for the course in a day. I discussed to my preacher and ask guidance from him. He just told me until you sense pain you are not in meditation. Once you enter in meditation faze will have no pains. I continued and followed his instructions. I experienced that when I continued more and more meditation I forgotten all pains and my body became lighter like a balloon. I continued to attend program and got good progress in meditation and resolved health issues like skin deices and muscular pains. I saw some of mediator got relief in migraine pain, ulcer in intestine and stomach. I was taking medicine for back pain also reduced and could stop after one month by continuing meditation practice daily.

When person try to be witness own thoughts, silence and meditation starts and become deeper and deeper which take you inward and where you can see true self and may communicate to superpower which provide you strength and peace of mind to your tired body.

Person become silent in afternoon sleep, night sleep and city also sleep, in deep sorrow, in full laughs, movement of the heavens and when living thing silent or avec nature and try to experience it's silence. You can see light of the joyless mind in silence, the lonely spirit in the troubled heart, work days worries where you see your true self as child or superpower.

Silence makes you holy, stillness and peaceful. It's where you are and shut the sense, sound, lights and merges the barrier of superpower, you become trouble free and you feel deeper peace of mind.

The purpose of the silence is not to see miracles which will distract you from the true purpose and keep away from your true self and superpower.

If you want to experience silence try to relax your body and keep open your mind remembering peaceful events you experienced, you cannot fight with thoughts and superpower so let it go and become tension free and feel superpower make your whole body relax, every nerve, every muscle, every cell relax and let it go. If you feel tension also relax and let it go, if you feel strained relax and let it go and this way you see your complete body relax and let it go and you will be fresh and relax.

You should be still when practice silence. Internal energy flow increase form universe to your body when your body is in still position, your mind is focused on one place and your internal energy concentrate at your mind focused point. If 2 out 3 things become steady your thoughts reduce, breath comes down and heart pulses comes down. Silence increases and you feel deeper meditation starts and you are in true self which takes you to ultimate peace. Your internal energy flow or bliss increases all the time you become calm and peaceful and feel your true self is part of superpower. Superpowe hears your innermost thoughts, faith, love and help you oneness during silence and thoughtless. When in thoughtless condition you ask to superpower anything becomes true. Remember that superpower's love has already encompassed the fulfillment of your needs.

You allow yourself thoughts positive, clear, sharp, still and hear superpower's voice in the silence and become peaceful without asking anything from superpower. You are blessed by superpower always and you also share these blessing to others.

Space and Silence

The gap is the silent space between two thoughts, gap between inhale and exhale, gap between musical rhythms or gap between two words in song.

Some people think it's really possible. If person concentrate it can be possible to hear and you will be silent at that point. I think superpower not created anything useless.

You should try to find out inner space by creating gaps in the stream of thinking without it becomes repetitive, uninspired, and empty of any creative spark.

You keep concentration on breath while meditation. It helps bringing space in your lives. You become conscious of your own breath and you are in present. Conscious breathing stops the process of thinking and remains aware and meditative.

Person wants peace should catch gap between two thoughts. If you can catch gap you will be silent and perform meditation and superpower support you and may you reach to self realization or to superpower. If you want to understand wisdom of your preacher is than be attentive to gap in between two words. You will enter in silence and ultimately in deep meditation. You may become good speaker later on by seeing gap and silence.

You develop inner silence, because you can give up the burden of your thoughts to superpower. There is much power to being in the Silence. Only in Silence, wisdom can arise. You remember that silence is so much more productive of wisdom and clarity in your thinking. You can develop silence without inner communication just observation and only observation. Your inner speech spins the delusions and cause of all the suffering. It makes you angry and for unwanted attachment to your friends and relatives. Its create guilt and depression.

You give unwanted burden to your mind with worry and fear. Once you become aware present moment there is no requirement of speech. You are completely in present moment and try to observe gap between your thoughts to have silence, peace and better meditation.

You observe attentively sharp mindfulness when one thought ends and before another thought starts, that is silence with awareness, it may be small and later on increases silence and also meditation increases. You can enjoy the silence. It's shy and if you talk disappeared at the same moment.

Your intension has tremendous power to organize and it lays effortless, continuous, obstruction free potential communication invisible to the visible. When you are thoughtless your volition for someone or yourself become true depending your progress and present position in meditation.

There is very thin barrier in between faith and blind faith. In all the part of world to many people slip in blind faith and ask God to complete their wish. I could not found proper word in English but it is conditional wish they put to God or superpower called" Baddha" in Indian local language. I try to explain with example, people goes to temple or religious place and ask God to give 100 gold biscuits and put condition that on receipt he will donate one biscuit to that temple or religious place. When I was in school I saw in my native place people asking God to give son or daughter, give good education or power of memory, buffalo give milk which stops, get bride for son, get money and so on and they offer something return to God if those fulfilled. They consider a God as agent, broker or commission agent. I want to say among these all wishes very few people could get their wish to be completed that were thoughtless when they asked to complete their wish from God and may be less than 1%. I saw this type of mentality in all the place and religious practices and encouraged to increase devotees and followers to individual authority. I once again sorry for hurting but keep in mind barrier in between faith and blind faith is very thin like a transparent curtain so be careful.

You can understand about gap by experience or by help of your preacher only. You don't bother for duration of gaps, initially few second enough and will grow as per your silence and meditation practices without any effort and ultimately your true self will be with superpower. You may not able to see gaps all the time but you have to leave up your all wishes than it will suddenly appears against you. Preacher says you have to leave up wish of self-realization or liberation and be witness one day you will get all the things without asking. You can enjoy silence and peace delightfully and become free.

If you listen song or music you will find gap between words or musical rhythms. This gap will take you to silence and then meditation. Music is a very good way to reach meditation and silence too. Music internally depends on silence, in some form or another to separate other period of sound and allow dynamics, melodies and rhythms to improve impact greater and more effective. You might have seen most music scores features rests we create period of silence. It takes person to contemplation or Samadhi. The person feels the effect of the previous notes and melodies and internally reflects on what they have heard. The silence does not abstract musical excellence but can amplify the sounds of instruments and vocals within a given musical composition.

One of the composers John Paynter said in his book that dramatic effect of silence has long been appreciated by composers. Some time general pause in the middle of the chorus have lightening and thunders and after the pause the music continues to the words gives same silence effects.

Tansen was mucian in Muslim king Akbar's time in India. He got very good position in silence and peace by music. He was playing music to make king happy all the time and unknowingly he had some symptoms burning body inside and he contacted Tana and Riri two sisters knew how to cool down inner side and progress in these circumstances.

In the 20Th, century composer discover further typical potential of silence in their music. These are used to teach experience of silence and meditation by some of the yogis. In jazz music "stop time" technique used to create silence effects.

Many religious prayers, practices, chantings are primary ways to learn mind activities or to control fickle nature and ultimately reach to silence, inner peace, meditation and contemplation or feretory. Ringing bell in temple also give good effect to concentrate in prayer of their God.

Some of the breathing exercise, Inhale(Puraka)-Retention(Antar Kumhaka)-Exhale(Rechaka)-Retention(Bahya Kumbhaka) cycle maintain and become silence and improve meditation, become thoughtless and get peace of mind.Retension may be increased as per Yoga teachers and it will improve better experience of silence and meditation. This is called Kumbhaka Pranayam; interested practiosner may refer astang yoga, pranayam or breathing exercises.

Kumbhaka Pranayam cycle explain in following graph. Retention should be followed as per yoga teacher or meditation preacher strictly.

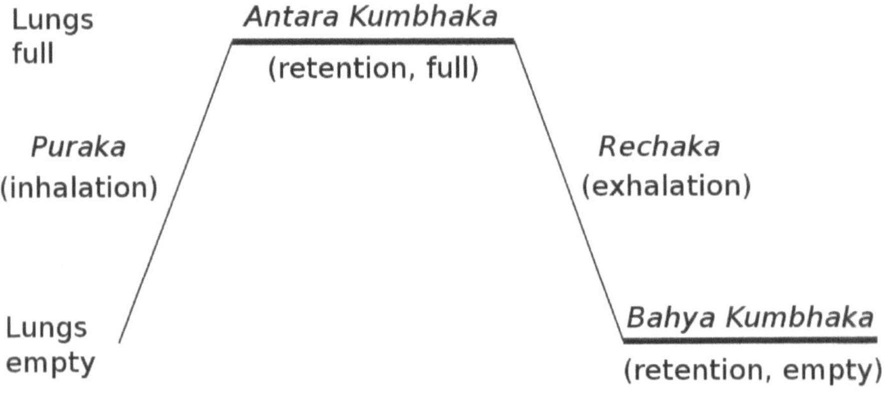

Benefits of Silence

There are so many physical or health benefits then spiritual of silence observed. It improves health, vitality and immune system. It takes away stress and makes you relax and recovered stress related problems. It increases vision to see with proper perspective with reason, clerity and understanding. It helps to overcome negative thoughts and hurt, guilt, depression, worry, anger, anxiety and tension. It helps you to control thoughts, to take right actions and decisions and save from troubles. It increases self awareness and gives opportunity to self-realization. It increases and open up your intuition and allow you deep thinking. It helps you to see with clarity and insight thinking. It makes you empathetic and understanding. It improves relationship to others. It helps to maintain harmony with people and world. It helps to become spiritual and meditative. It takes you to deeper parts or subconscious mind. Silence keeps away from noise and hence additional stress.

Its control stress and anxiety, Improve sleep pattern, Reduce inflammation, improve in irritable bowel syndrome and post-traumatic stress disorder and fibromyalgia.

It also reduces anxiety disorder, such as phobias paranoid thoughts, obsessive compulsive behaviors and panic attacks. It reduces job related anxiety in working group. Its decrease depression, improve mood, improve mind wandering and warrying, may reduce age related memory loss, generate kindness, may help fight addictions, helps to control various pains and decrease blood pressure.

It Improve memory, stimulate brain growth by creating new cells, improve stress related issues, fight insomnia and improve sleep related problems, reduce heart problems, increase courage, inner strength, increase confidence, transcends all understanding.

It renews souls, reminds that life will still go on without anyone, clears the problems of life and mind for wise decision making and planning and breaks the power of hurry, remove addiction to a "have to do" mentality.

It keeps away noise of TV, music and mobile, email, text, call and technology's magnetic fields. It gives space to think, act and play with our mind and very healthy for our physical and mental wellbeing, bust body's immune system, promote good hormone regulation and interaction of bodily hormone related systems, prevent plaque formation in arteries and increase sensitivity to flow of life force.

Silence and Meditation

You keep in mind that meditation will be in silence and can be practice by learning from preacher or experienced person. You should try to do chant mantras or good thoughts which are for beginners and should not continue for all the time.

When we put our kids to junior, senior kitten garden school and primary school they try to teach counting 1-100 numbers by balls but later on they remember numbers and leave up balls. You can chant mantra or good thoughts in first few days and leave up that practice, try to become thoughtless and be witness of thoughts.

From thousands of years silent meditation was reserved people who leave up family and loved one called Renunciation but it's available through various organization to all kind and group of people now a days.

You should be patience if want to learn silence, progress in meditation and have peace of mind. There is proverb you cannot get crop of mango in hurriedly.

You should be diligent to get silence and meditation. Once you have it you think to reduce time for same but you may miss out the vast benefits of consistent meditation. You should continue it when you feel calmness and try to make deeper and clear. You feel it comes and go so be preserved and follow continuously.

You try to do meditation everyday will help you to be silent and better one in daily tasks so spare time from your busy schedule. You try to start this practice as an integral part of your daily routine like other daily activities than you develop the mental space to be more direct, focused and efficient for the rest of day.

Your sleep will reduce by meditation some time so do not be in panic and cut down sleeping time in day time. You will feel fresh all the day and active for the work without hurting your efficiency.

You will be contented by meditation but your feeling may vary and not same all the day. You should continue meditation one day you will have bliss and your mediation definitely improves. You try to observe feelings without any affection or prejudice and continue the meditation practice one day you will be master and definitely find your goal.

Vipassana meditation brought back in India from 1969 from Burma by Shri Satyaprakash Goyankaji. It's to be practiced avec complete silence. You don't have to stop thoughts forcefully. You have to observe sensation. You should be in present and try to keep away from past and future. Don't try to change anything like thoughts, emotions, and feelings but just observe and accept. You should see your mind like sky and thoughts are like cloud, slowly thoughts go away like clouds and mind will become like clear sky. It's teaching to be in mindfulness of breathing and sensation by utilizing feelings and actions. You are not allowed to do other meditation practice or yoga, Tai, chi, aerobics along it. Keep away bad habits like smoking, drugs or alcohol. Don't speak with people and avoid direct eye contacts. You should avoid writing instructions, listening to music, reading or using mobile, radio and television.

You remember in mind means words, true self means silence. Words stored in unconscious mind and come out when you do meditation, empty out and you become silent. It will be always with you. You can say its true self and your internal quality so don't forget accumulation of words but do not participate and be witness.It may go to unconscious mind. You can say silence is meditation and practice to shift the attention from words into silence and it's remaining with you all the time.

You should make your mind like still water in which you can see your image clearly and like that true self see super power and experience deep silence and meditation where more powerful communication is taking place in deeper awareness.

Your awareness that exists beyond world allows your direct experience to complete fresh. It more make receptive you to this awareness,more quickly language and thought are analyzed for usefulness and released where more and more consistenly,as it become stronger in its habits. It dissolves barriers between us and other. Some person feel uncomfortable with silence, they normally cannot become thoughtless very easily.

Remember that very sensitive person cannot adjust with worldly people but meditation can make them comfortable, make silent and happy. When you have pains become aware and continue meditation on it and in pleasure use it as drowning or forgetfulness and do meditation.

You experience of zeal in meditation or Samadhi by becoming one with rhythm of universe and allow your true self merge in it and enjoy silence, meditation and peace.

Your senses tell you about world but inner sense something about yourself and superpower, if you can find out inner sense than you can merge to superpower and have peace of mind.

You should surrender to reality and don't fight otherwise those will create conflict cause wondering mind and you will be loser. Your ego disappears and become awareness of which always should be there to have enter in silence and deep meditation.

If you want love you should start to give your love to others. If you want bliss you try to share your bliss to others. If you think flowers showers in your home than you should showers those to other people's home. This is only way you can share compassions and enter to silence and meditation.

You have to do the entire thing with awareness like eat, love, walk, doing work or 24 hours daily work what you do, superpower bliss showers to you which will take you to silence and meditation.

When meditation grows inside you, your desire come down and you become contented whatever you have. You will have no desire means you are close to superpower and anytime you will merge yourself in it. There is nothing to get in this worldly life except it.

When you forget mind, thoughts and witness them than you experience meditation, silence and peace of mind. Your internal energy starts flowing in every part of bodies and addition in it starts flowing from universe continuously make you sunk yourself in silence, meditation and peace.

Although words are mainly intended to form bridges of communication, they often have the opposite effect. Many people use words simply to fill the void that they feel inside themselves. They are uncomfortable with silence, and so they chatter. They hope to connect with others, but often they should avoid having better experience of silence and meditation.

I learn if we are sad to the world, the world will sad to us but we smile to the world, the world smile to us. I can control emotions and feeling and possibly keep away anger. I became calm after completing the course. I learnt negative emotion come from me, not from others. I became more aware and thoughtful. I came out from worries and stress. I understand to go on the way of life without bothering. I understand to forgive myself and others. I learnt to enjoy owness.I learnt to wait for good thing to happen in my life not to worry for future which is not in my hand. I learn to think peacefully and not hurriedly. I am able to accept happenings in present and avoid all past memory because nothing can be changed.

If you meet a silent person, preacher their wave enters to you. The primenister of India met priest once. She asked some questions and listen replies. She left the place and came to her plane. One of journalist surprised and asked her what's happened by seeing her calmness. She replied it was nice meeting but still my inner soul instructing me to remain silent.

Some meditation practice teach to chant good thoughts or mantras while meditation which cannot be consider silence because person is with good thoughts and try to push negative thoughts. It may take person in silence or thoughtless condition over a period.

Same way lots of religious persons doing prayers, singing religious songs, performing religious dance, listening storyline, discourse and philosophical talks are also consider good thoughts which keeps away from negative thoughts but not in silence. Silence is only way to reach meditation and have peace of mind. Other than it are longer ways to reach final destination said self realization or God.

Every religions or preachers described or arranged different ways to reach silence. In one of the Indian book 112 methods are described to perform meditation and attain silence or peace. If person continue by any method or way shown by preacher and do the practice he will be in meditation. If they are in trouble superpower send good guide or Wiseman to complete their wish or required good actions.

In Serpentine or Kundalini meditation people follow silence and do meditation by seeing thoughts without involve them or participate them. It's called be witness avec thoughts. Slowly thought frequency comes down and quality of meditation improves. In this meditation breathing, blood pressure, heart pulse comes down as improving silence and meditation. Person become calm and ultimately reach to self realization and contemplation. This is very old technique followed in India and some other countries.

Vipassana is also thoughtless method and teach to see sensation on body for less than one minute at one place and move mind to other place of body. Mind to not become rigid and start wondering in this method.

Technically both methods have slight difference which I will try to explain by example. We keep overhead tank on our roof and maintain level in it. There are practice to provide float switch and it gives signal to stop motor when tank become full or set level. If not float switch person has to take care and stop motor when he feels level is achieved in tank. The first method of float switch is compared with serpentine method of meditation because practitioner has to focus mind on one place, allow superpower to do rest of the thing and be witness of thoughts. Second method have no float switch is like Vipassana method practitioner has to decide and move mind place to place. Serpentine method is ancient method and Vipassana method suggested by Buddha before 2600 years ago. Both methods can be considered thoughtless meditation and Vipassana 10 days course followed with silence.

Various Religions and Meditation

Various religious group's priests have different practices. Some were believe to say storyline or discourse after taking food or donation. They taught about good cheracters, enjoyment and control over bad habits. They believe they should return 10 times what they got from family who donate food to them. Some give just blessing "be happy".

Some group think not to speak is silence and other think speak for good cause is also silence. Internal thoughtless is silence.

If person wants too many things and ambitious will never become silent. If your requirements minimum and practice for meditation you may enter in it with less problems and you can get silence and peace. When unnecessary thoughts come down peace or silence starts but if remain continue mind will remain disturbed and no silence or peace in mind.

If you reach silence, peace and talk or speak something for good cause mind remains calm because internal silence or peace and bliss continuously flows to you. Normally foolish people talks too much cannot get silence or peace. Wise people speak some time for good cause their peace not disturbed much and regain previous condition immediately. They remain silent when they do not talk and no one requires their help.

Wise people want to share what they got and for that they speak to people sometime. Sharing for betterment of mankind is always good. I saw when Vipassana course complete all participants have to share 10% what they got while 10 -45 days course to others were not there and universal animals and insects.

If you read this book and like something. You should share to your friends and others. Whatever you do well for others, retune bake to you more and more in multiple times is universal law. Buddha said lot of people knows but they are not able to practice and they have so many luxury in life but want silence and peace which never be possible. If person wants silence and peace he has to leave up all desires. If you want to get truth be empty. Silence is positive so you should not mix up negative with it otherwise silence will go away. Share others. Sometime person reach to truth but don't want to share others. They think its annoyance to share others. They think we got diamond why to give others. Person wandering to get wealth.

When child born having no boundaries of religions. Those taught by different level of society, fed by family, sourrounding and society. Peaceful and silent soul becomes disturbed and violent by these types of boundaries and various ideas.

If you use thousands of words useless you become disturbed but you use one word useful you will become silent. You should think before you speak.

If you kill or hurt somebody, stealing some one's properly, sexual misconduct, laying and intoxication are not good qualities so keep away to improve silence and meditation. These are requirement who want to do Vipassana course for 10 days or longer. It disturb mind after doing such activities and takes long time to cool down mind. If you throw stone in dirty pond water so pond disturbs, it looks dirty and cannot see through it. When it settled after some time it looks clean same way person can disturbed and mind wandering after doing above mentioned 5 activities.

One person named Anguliman in India was so disturbed by mind and decided to kill 1000 persons. He killed 999 persons and waiting one person to pass by that forest. People were so afraid and stop to go in that forest. One day Buddha was passing to that forest. People requested not to go there but he continued and met that violent man. He also told Buddha to go away otherwise he will kill him. Buddha told him to break one branch of tree and he did it. Buddha told now you fix back that branch to tree again. He told it's not possible to fix back. He advises if you cannot fix back why you should break. He asked Buddha can you fix it? Buddha said I always do work for fixing and he became disciple of Buddha. His mind became calm and all disturbances gone away. He became very good follower of Buddha and passed his life peacefully. This shows how disturbed minded person can be changed in presence whose thoughts positive and full of internal energy.

You can say in spiritual meaning of meditation is not process of mind but spirit. There are two stage concentration and contemplation. People gather attention with devotion in superpower or God and raising it to one of the focal center in body. People know as single eye, eye of the soul, third eye or tenth door as per their beliefs. Once "eye of soul" or inner eyes awaken the human soul may contemplate the divine light of superpower or God and believed it's as light. There is religious belief that human soul also has inner ear with which it can tune into The Devine power or universe vibrations. Physical body consider house for soul. Person should know oneself and later on Divinity and find out about existence and true self which is divine spirit is called one of spiritual nature. The contemplating the inner Light and listening inner sound by the grace of superpower is meditation. The human soul to have the ability to "see" and "hear" is called Holy Ghost or Holy Spirit.

Person should follow the path with a calm and peaceful spirit. You should completely surrender to superpower or preacher in meditation for better result. Its water and bread of life discussed in Scriptures.

You should do meditation daily with calm, love, leave up discouragement, being optimist, faith, joy, cheers will allow energies upward which gather at focal center and take to the superpower.

The Light and Sound within takes person to superpower. The instructions are not available in religious literatures as discussed and passed verbally by religious preachers.

Various religious masters gave a double message for common public and chosen disciples. Their idea to discussed inner peace and true self subject for better understanding people first and common public later on when they develop them self and improve understanding power. I think they were correct as Master degree or doctorate degree eligibility is after completion bachelor degree given now a day also.

The qualities comes with Divinity are light, love,life, grasped through experience and reach to truth which everything described or closed in formula may not be attributed to the Divinity. The masters not wants person to prisoners of any exterior practice which is only primary level. Truth with love and the soul can be experienced like a sea of shower or bliss, knowledge and peace. The divine light, soul and superpower are opens road to high-test knowledge of true self and ego may be obstruction to it.

The term "Master" used in spirituality from long time in the world but if restricted by some religious can read as preacher.

The main religions like Hinduism, Buddhism, Judaism, Christianity and Islam meditation plays a part to greater or lesser degrees depending up on individuals liking. All the practices of meditation some differences are there but an ultimate goal is to reach super power, silence and peace of mind.

Meditation in Hinduism:

There is great role of meditation in every aspect of Indian spiritual life depending up on individual practitioner's path and their preacher's selected method. The term Hindu means different groups settled in Hindustan and called India during British rule.

India is a highly diverse country with a long history that has many interwoven traditions, including Buddhism. There are various religion books in which meditation subjects discussed by masters and have unique contribution to spiritual practice. The Patanjali Eight Limbs of Yoga is most popular guide line to meditation practitioners. The brief description is as under.

Yamas and its complements, Niyamas represent various right living or ethical rules.

1-Yamas: There are five social ethics.

- Ahinsa-non violence in action, speech and thoughts.

- Satyam-truthfulness in intension and remain highest in truth.

- Asteya: Not to steal somebody's thing.

- Brahamcharya: One should have divine conduct, celibate when single and faithful to partner when married.

- Aparigraha: One should avoid accumulating things not useful and don't desire things belong to others.

2-Niyamas: Those are the five personal ethics.

- Saucha: One should maintain cleanliness of the body and mind.

- Santosha: One should have contentment; remain happy in whatever available thing with someone.

- Tapas: One should maintain austerity and self-discipline.

- Swadhyaya: One should study of the self and abiding in the self.

- Ishwarapranidhana: One should have surrender to God and honoring the Devine superpower.

3-Asanas: Seat for yoga or meditation and seating position.

4-Pranayams: Proper regulation of prana through certain breathing techniques.

5-Pratayahara: One should take the senses inwards.

6-Dharana: One should focus on one point while meditation.

7-Dhyana: One should practice meditation

8-Samadhi: It is the highest state of consciousness when progressing in meditation.

Those want to know more should refer Patanjali Yoga Sutras.

There are about 112 different meditation practices described in Bhairavtantra Vigyan book and their master teaching to their disciples so someone should not be confused by reading this book but catch whatever suit to them and continue their practice.

Meditation in Buddhism:

Buddha identified eight principles (The Noble Eightfold Path) that develop the fully realized state of a person; right view, right resolve, right speech, right conduct, right livelihood, right effort, right awareness, right meditation.Vipassan,to look inward is popular meditation practice with 10 days silence and meditation. There are centers available all over the world.

Meditation in Judaism:

In the Hebrew language Qabalah is used to receive and to show. Those are metaphysical doctrine and philosophy, the tradition within a tradition of Qabalah is a symbolic code designed to further practitioner's spiritual development and growth.

Students of the Qabalah transform their essential inner natures with the essential external Nature, by internalizing symbols and gradually absorbing their characteristics through meditation. The central symbol of Qabalah is a cosmogram. The Tree Of Life (Otz Chim) composed of eleven spheres (sephiroth), one of which is hidden, interconnected by twenty two pathways. Each sephora bears a different name of God, representing different aspects of the divine. They are crown, wisdom, understanding, knowledge, severity, mercy, beauty, victory, glory, foundation, and kingdom. Symbols are assigned to each sephira including title, name, image, color, and number.

Meditation awakens the higher faculties of the individuals, transcending reason, and bringing the symbols to life.

Meditation in Christianity:

Christian forms of meditation have a long history, though not all practices are accepted universally in the all churches (including but not limited to Orthodox, Catholic, Lutheran, Baptist, Protestant, Episcopalian, Quaker, Shaker, and Gnostic). The Desert Fathers, early hermits who established the basis for the Christian withdrawn life either individually or in groups, used repeated prayer, either spoken or sung, with synchronized breathing to internalize the spiritual truths contained within them. The Eastern Orthodox traditions practice creating and using icons as a focus for meditation. The Jesuit traditions use visualization and imagination to respond in a deeply felt personal way to scenes from the life of Christ (including Nativity, Passion, Crucifixion, and Resurrection) and internalized the lessons that can be found within them. The simplest and most universal form of Christian meditation can be found in the practice of repeating prayers, either individually, together, or in a cycle.

Whether expressed through song, prayer, study or contemplation, focus is generally directed first towards the heart, producing a deeply felt understanding that suffuses the whole being.

Meditation in Islam:

Rooted in the Koran and the teachings of Muhammad, Islam's mystical path Sufism includes commentaries by masters and teachings from a wide range of esoteric traditions including the Zoroastrian, the Hermetic, and the Pythagoreans. It is further supplemented by a rich literary tradition that emphasizes poetry, allegory, and symbolic story. The arts reveal universal principles and everyday activities become vehicles for meditation,writing, calligraphy, geometry, architecture, dance, weaving, etc. Everything is considered sacred and unity is expressed everywhere.

The pupil teacher relationship is central to Sufi spiritual practice; only those who have been recognized by previous masters as masters (a chain that goes back to the prophet) have the authority to initiate pupils. Masters dictate meditation practices, which can vary substantially in the final form they take. The aim of meditation (fikr) is to prevent the mind from going astray while the heart is focuses on God. The spoken word (prayer, chant, song) is heavily emphasized as an active invocation of God through repetition of the Holy Names (zikr).

Meditation in Other Religions:

Many other spiritual traditions have practices that are identical in form and function to these practices and they offer many more. How similar these divergent practices are to meditation is often a matter of degree. The discussion of how similar some of these practices are is useful. While not unrelated, trance states, often involving a loss of self-awareness can be distinctly different. Similarly, altered states of mind induced by chemical agents can be similar in many ways but are also distinctly different in others. Meditation rarely, if ever, involves a loss of self-awareness or control; quite the opposite, it almost always heightens both.

Despite the fact that meditation can take many forms, universal principles can be found in all systems. The whole being (body, mind, and emotion) is actively applied, through a variety of focus points, to develop awareness, insight, and transformation. Normally focus point, chanting is different for various practices but ultimate goal remains to get peace of mind and reach to the superpower.

"We need to find God, and he cannot be found in noise and restlessness. God is the friend of silence. See how nature-trees, flowers, grass-grows in silence, see the stars, the moon and the sun, how they move in silence. We need silence to be able to touch soul"-Mother Teresa

First of all I thanks to Mother Teresa for her beautiful quote. Silence flows in nature so ancient yogis preferred to pass their time for meditation in forest, caves, bank of river or seashore. They have experienced the internal flows of silence so they can share to people those want and approach to them. If you walk on grass berfooted, dip your legs in the river or sea water, touch to the trees, take bath in river, pond or sea you will get freshness. They take all the negative vibrations or energy and allow passing positive vibrations or energy from universe or bliss from superpower these ultimately increase your silence and improve meditation quality and peace of mind. Yogis always advise to people to pass their time avec nature and nature's innocent creation.

If you are in countries where houses are made out from wood it's possible that your internal energy may not ground. You may get spark when you touch to shining handle of door or window or machines and utensils made out of metals which can transmit electricity. One of my coworker in Yemen opening the door of our wooden container office and touching brass handle I saw he was experiencing spark. If you feel same problem walk on grass barefooted, dip your legs in the river or sea water, touch to the trees, take bath in river, home, bath tub, pond or sea.

People search for God or superpower from thousands of years but very few have experienced. One of the Indian saints explained very nicely with example which I will like to describe here.Kasturi is obtained from the rectal (Naval) of Musk deer. It is used in making perfumes, incenses as well as in medicine makings. It's in Navel of Musk deer but it search whole life in grass, ground or forest but never look inside likewise supper power sleeping inside person's body but we search out side and never see inward. Silence will be inward not in outer world.

If you go to listen storyline, narrative or discourse you should be thoughtless to understand but they creates dispute and you cannot understand complete meaning.Try to listen preachers heartfully.If you listen by brain it makes debate and disturb you. These persons experience silence and its flow their inner soul so if you listen by your heart silence will directly flow to your heart and you are the luckiest person so try to hear them very deeply and artfully without any prejudice or doubt. If you know theory of philosophy but it will never take you to truth. Highly positioned people have higher ego and that only can be broken by preacher. We get peace if we hear the words of saint or preacher and seat closely. Silence flow starts in our inner soul which gives us experience of peace.

We can summaries that nature, saint or preacher can give us flow of positive energy and thus silence. We can experience peace and deep meditation. Person has to do meditation everyday 20 minutes to 3 hours a day to make up and maintain internal energy and peace.

Our preacher advises us to gather one place once a week or more and do meditation in group. These give energy flow or silence flow and peace to us and make us rich with positive energy. Some religious they gathered for prayer at one place have same idea. The constructions of temple,churche or religious building are constructed such a way so that maximum positive energy or bliss enter to the building from highest point of dome and participant benefited maximum. I always experience good energy flow when I visit Saint Josef Church in Montreal which is having highest dome and surrounded by garden and forest.

Once again I remind this positive energy or bliss we discussed is found in every religious places or meditation halls. The quantity of richness level depends up on so many circumstances. It's always to go and participate where your mind feel silence and peace without any prejudice. I have practice wherever I feel positive energy and I didn't saw any difference in energy levels. I like you to try and understand participate such gatherings heartfully and cheerfully to enrich your energy level and peace.

Thoughts Observation and Peace

The flow of consciousness we only experience one mental event at a time as a fast moving mind stream. These events are also described as being influenced by attachments and past conditioning and other various laws of universe. Some scientist says its illusion and not real as such it seen. Thoughts are like flowing water of river as they come and go, more we let them allow freely flow bigger the stream becomes. Thoughts can be reduced by seeing and be witness and allow silence and hence peace to inner mind. This is just like river water also blocks or constructing dam on the river to stop flow. We can experience thoughts by being aware of it also if we witness, frquency of thoughts reduced. More we aware of our thoughts more silence attract towards us and we experience deeper peace and meditation.

I saw old age people may be 70+ years sitting on the bench of park or street. They go on talking about politics normally they watched on television or heard on radio or read in news paper. I don't see a single talk can give them peace or silence but they want to be empty out mind or stored memory and want to be happy. On the other end who hears such a talk are getting bored or sometime participate slightly to make show that they understood. Some people talk about their family problem, health problem, their beliefs but all want to be empty out their mind with someone. May be silence not allowing them seat peacefully. I saw these types of people to learn how to be silent, get peace or do meditation. They leave up course within 3-4 days. They lost their patience. Silence becomes effective if someone practice with patience can get and able to reduce their thoughts. Once thoughts come down attain meditation. Some time people want everything in very short time or they trained their mind to go on talking and empty out their garbage to others that is why silence makes them uncomfortable. I think those who want silence or peace should come out from dumping this type of garbage in their mind by media or surroundings. If their talks and thoughts are unguarded or meaningless harm them more than their enemy and other listeners too.

People go to hear storyline but do not hear carefully. They understand mad for bad and confused themselves. If they listened heartfully, with love than silence flows to their mind and they may be able to stop wandering their mind and completely understand what storyline is. If they change themselves they understand or they grow in real term. They need to change their methods; habits if they want silence and peace because persons shaped as per their thoughts and become what they think.

One student wants to do meditation so went to one yogi. Yogi told you do not have to allow thought of monkey in your mind and come to me after one week. Student gone back home and try to read books. Thoughts of monkey came to his mind. He tried to sleep he got thoughts of monkey came to his mind. He was trying to keep away thoughts of monkey but it was all the time come to his mind. He tired and gone to yogi and told I don't want to learn meditation but please keep away thoughts of monkey from my mind. Yogi shows one pole and told that student to climb up to that pole and come down from it and continue doing. Yogi called him at the end of day and asked him is thoughts of monkey in your mind? Student said no, I didn't get thought of monkey in my mind.

Moral of this story is that which thought you want to push out from your mind comes again and again. If you keep your mind engaged that thought remains away from your mind.

It is discussed in Indian philosophical books that it's very difficult to control or engage mind. If you can control flow of wind or catch air than control mind. Its 5000 years back thoughts but now a day person invented compressor which compresses air or gases and fill up in cylinders. That time also superpower replied that by practice and take out your mind from wishes, pains and troubles and just be witness it's possible.

There are many practices to control thoughts and allow silence to enter to mind and become peaceful. One is not to participate in the thoughts and just observe them and be witness. Other thing to engage in activity such to move on body and see what happening or getting sensation on the body. So many ways are shown by Indian yogis like chanting name of God, remembering good qualities of God or seeing breath and chanting. These all not allowing being thoughtless but engaging you with good thoughts or activities.

Its observed more or less by these methods person can reduce frequency of thoughts and allowing silence to enter in mind and be peaceful or meditative.

When there is no-I means forget ego than thoughts stops and silence starts. It's in person's mind. It's permanent and benefit to humanity. The consciousness is with silence is aim of peace lover. Person can say silent "I" is God, superpower, Soul, flowing positive energy flow or ancient world. It's also described in Gayatri Mantra in Rig-Veda that God is "Pranswarup" can say flowing positive energy inward. The experience of silence is perfect knowledge. It's very difficult to explain silence in words but just can be experienced. It's helpful for doing meditation. Person's own attention is silence and nothing else. It' said that your preacher is main source of silence or positive energy. Silence takes person to liberation, keep away from all the worries and pains if ego also vanished. Person who realized silence is more powerful and can send vibration or spiritual waves from remote place to others also. Some time person fails to understand conversation several years can be known instantly by silence. Silence purifies someone by every way. Some time great books fails to explain can be understood by silence in no time. Silence means not navigation of activity. Superpower and liberated soul are routed in silence and work remotely without speech. True nature of person is egoless silence. Person can reach to someone's heart by silence only. Silence is the profound truth of Vedanta and all religions ends up in it. Person is not thinking or knowing anything in silence except oneness. In the fullness of silence there is only consciousness without any thoughts. Person experience bliss in silence is not possible to get in anywhere. Person in silence feel that conscious is doing everything not body. Silence gives feeling of young forever. Silence is creating sense of fullness. When silence rise and ego ends up. It is the axis of everything. Person sunk in the ocean of silence when one is at the top of consciousness. From silence came thought, from thought the ego, and from ego, speech. So if speech is so effective than how much more effective source of all of them silence is? Practicing silence, Self-enquiry and to remain in is true mental worship. Person should believe superpower or preacher as lord till attain liberation. Person who remains always is wise and better understanding. You should enthrone the Lord upon the seat of the Heart and keep the whole mind at the feet and do worship is a best worship. The inner silence is self-surrender that live without the sense of ego. Subjugation of the mind is meditation. Silence is permanent and benefits the whole of humanity. Silence is better than oral lectures. State of happiness is silence through heart and to forget "I am this body "The silence of self which shines through pure mind is gateway of liberation. You attend unceasingly and with a fully concentrated mind to self, which is the non-dual perfect reality, alone is the pure Supreme silence. Shiva (the Self), are those who are soaked in the perfect and natural state of silence and removed the "I"-sense. Superpower or God is the egoless self. You should remain silent and give up all the anxieties of mind is best. You should know that silence – which is the perfect knowledge of the form of self and which shines within when the ego reaches the Heart by rejecting all the juggleries of thoughts. If the noise of thoughts not stops silence is not attain. Keep your mind still you will get spiritual help and power of self will be experienced. The wave of self will pervade everywhere and you will be silent.

Preacher can send waves of internal energy or spiritual influence which can reach too many people even if he seat far away maintaining silence and send messages without uttering single word. If necessary he can use others as instruments. Some time person who sits in a holy presence and goes away after some time with his outlook on life totally changed. Silent initiation changes the hearts of all is the best one.Superpower, grace and preacher are helping same way. Silence is the most potent form of work. However vast and emphatic the scriptures may be fail in their effect, silence is ever speaking. It is a perennial flow of language, which is interrupted by speaking. These words I am speaking obstruct that mute.

Person attains silence and become kind, loving and helpful to others. He thinks betterment and necessicity of others also. If person practice for seven days his face glowing and aura improve. During silence you are alone in peace. We clean our utensils everyday like we should do meditation also every day. When person is sick he should take rest and proper sleep so his internal energy increases and help to recover and medicine also works. If he can remain silence more and more internal energy enters and become healthy.

Normally person become sick his internal energy level comes down. He should try to remain in contact of person having higher level of internal energy. He can seat in front of sunlight also helps.

He can take natural fresh foods. He can walk in garden or green grass. Hospital many patient visits so energy level remains lower.

Person's blood Ph becomes acidic during sickness. He has to try to make it basic. He can take milk or boil legumes which can helps. If possible walking, light exercises or deep breathing should be done. You can cut down processed foods. Consume containing vitamin B such as whole grains, bananas, beans and light meals. Increase fiber intake such as fruits and vegetables may also help.

Silence and Samadhi

The Indian sage Patanjali has taught us systematic path to reach higher consciousness or awaken the mind to its true self and Samadhi. Patanjali's Eight Limbs of Yoga is a very famous book and interested person can refer it. I have discussed in brief in earlier chapter.

Samadhi state can be defined dormant position with awareness. During sleep we are not aware what is happening around us so it's not Samadhi state. Silence position if there are no waves or dream but thoughtless condition is called Samadhi state. You are entering deeper in your mind and enjoying the condition. You may realize that you are very near to truth. You should not listen what others say but listen internal voice and be happy. Normally person believes what others say and ignore internal voice and face too many problems in life. If mob say certain leader is very good all believe but actually that's not true because mob itself is creation of the leader for publicity. Never be happy or upset by others words.

When I was studying in Master of Science class our professor was advising it's useless to continue master course. If you get job join because there will be same job you have to do later on. Most of the students tried to search job and joined. The professor was breaking the confidence of the students and turning them to search job. If he had given good advice like after completing course you can do doctor degree or go to start your factory some of students could do it. You will get such persons every steps of life so be confident and hear your inner voice and follow it.

I learnt about Thomas Alva Edison that he was not brilliant student. His teacher called his mother and said your son can not continue this school. His mother took out him from the school and made arrangement to continued his studies at home or other school. He became scientist later on and find out electric bulb. It means what others say is not correct. You should be confident and follower of your inner soul. Keep in mind you are the best judge for yourself

Samadhi state is a highest achievement of meditation when all the thoughts stops and you are in deeper silence and with your true self and nothing else. Most of the people become silent and not able to describe experience of that position which I came to know from the book of Indian yogi Ramakrishna Paramhansa. He was not able to speak after crossing throat chakra when asked their disciples to know what is happening in Samadhi state.

It is described in Vedas that everything in world has awareness. Mountains, trees, animals, sea, rivers and humans have awareness but humans have power for self awareness. Animal never ask "Who am I?" So every human can reach to state of Samadhi and experience silence, thoughtless condition and peace of mind. The grace of preacher helps and supports every stage to achieve this goal. Person will get good qualities like love, kindness, helping to others, faithfulness and leave up all bad qualities if someone experience state of Samadhi.

Until your silence not break up some time thoughts come but you remain witness of them and you remain in silence. If a person throw stone to pond water or animal enter to pond water get disturbs and seen dirty. When stone settle down to bottom and animal comes out from the pond, dirt settle down and its look clear. When you reach to inner peace, your speech become attractive, holy and your personality become such that people come and like to stay with you because your mind become clean as like settled water of pond. They also ask and expect help for solving their issues. It's better if you do without any reward and nature also helps you for the same cause. Some person misuse this power and their progress slow down or stop. People enjoy your company and your speech and slowly they like to follow your advice.

In reality person who experience silence and peace become silent. Person who are greedy, ambitious and wants benefits from people speak too much which harm to people and society. It's better if person who experienced silence should speak and share experience to others but some of them become silent keep away from the society. Superpower also wants that he speak to others because other gets benefit by his speech. Buddha shared his knowledge for betterment of mankind up to 80 years of his life but others didn't.

Person who reached to state of Samadhi and inner peace are lucky but share to someone may be more useful for society as discussed earlier.

We should remember and reach to inner peace and silence and share to maximum people so they also learn and follow the path of silence. Stored water always gives bad smell so be like flowing water and share to others. Nature also helps such person for sharing his peace. Person who reached to silence and peace have special divine lights in their eyes which attract all people and get benefit from them. All the time positive energy flowing outward and surroundings and all are getting benefits who are nearby. They distribute all without seeing anything. Sometime outer world say person who reach to silence and peace is mad because he share without any expection. Wroldly people give something and need something. When person reach to silence and peace his ego becomes zero and he can see his death so some people afraid and leave up this path. Many people tried but few people reach to that goal.

Person should try to merge senses in mind, mind to intelligence, intelligence to soul and then true self-soul merge to contemplation and contemplation to merge to superpower. Finally true self and superpower becomes one so there is no barrier in between. Now your mind flooded with unlimited thoughts but slowly you try to be silent one by one thought comes down and you will experience silence, peace and ultimate truth superpower. Meditation is a path of mind and true self and door to reach superpower.

There is different level of state of Samadhi which is very difficult to explain by words but you can refer in Patanjali Eight Limbs of Yoga. I am trying to explain whatever I know.

There are two types of Samadhi as per Patanjali, Samprajnata Samadhi with higher knowledge which occurs through the absorption of the mind into object. Asamprajnata Samadhi-"beyond higher knowledge" a very high stage in which there in no object of concentration, without practitioner's consciousness.

Samadhi state also known as Transcendence is a state where the frequency of brain is beyond zero and separate body from the soul. The Samadhi means bring together or unification of mind where person's karma burns out as per Hinduism.

Samadhi is the matter of soul, all the chakras should be clean and a state of oneness acchived.Its state practitioner identity of his soul as spirit and experience of supercoscious perception. It can be experience for 30 seconds to two minutes. I read long back masters experience many days without food and water too.

It's an equal state of consciousness where all aspects of one's being are merged, physical, spiritual, mental and emotional. Someone get shower of bliss, super enlightenment or self-realization.

Samadhi is "total self-collectedness" in Indian religion, and particularly in Hinduism and Buddhism, the highest state of mental concentration that a person can achieve while still bound to the body and which unites someone with the highest reality.

Bliss is a state of unity, transcendence, completeness, knowingness, wholeness, and uplifted consciousness; it is a feeling of oneness and connection with all of creation. Bliss is never boring; it feels ever new, expansive, and infinite.

You can get complete rest in silence and meditation and become thrice fresh than sleep. You are in conscious rest where you are in deepest inner self withought any thoughts and with true self or superpower is state of Samadhi.

I read about four types of Samadhi:

Vitarkanugama Samadhi is a state of silence, calm attained by logical reasoning.

Vicharanugama Samadhi is the same state where thoughts exist but not disturbing oneself.

Anandnugama Samadhi is a state in which someone showered by bliss from superpower and enjoys silence and peace of mind.

Asmitanugama Samadhi is inner most true self experience after that someone wants nothing.

It is mentioned in Patanjali Yog Sutra that some person feel deep rest naturally without any additional efforts. This may be the results of previous incarnation practices or soul's uplifted position. I read Raman Maharishi achieved state of Samadhi without any master's help in India. This type of person rarely available who doesn't need help of preacher or master.

It's observed some people get the state of Samadhi without any efforts may be due to past incarnation achievement, karmas or samskaras but most of the people have to practice under the guidance of masters and continue for long time to reach state of Samadhi.

Vitarkanugama Samadhi is state where suddenly someone realized consciousness about the truth like prince Siddhartha's case happened and later on he became Buddha. Someone can understand truth and real meaning of the creation of everything.

Some time person experience disturbing thoughts not with closed eyes but open eyes also and have capacity to disturb others also from remote place.

Vicharanugama Samadhi is a state of Samadhi someone behaves like outsider with thoughts say be witness and not disturbed by thoughts. The various thoughts in the form of smells, lights, visions, tastes and sounds which come to one as an experience during meditation. Some practitioner got smell of sandalwood which I saw.

Anandanugama Samadhi is blissful state of Samadhi where mind and consciousness are at upper level but sometime experience overwhelming feeling of great happiness or joyful excitement and endless bliss.

Asmitanugama Samadhi is a state of Samadhi where you lose track who are you or where are you and forget everything yourself and around you.

In some cases mind merge with object even if sound where there is no meditation or meditator and the thinker and thoughts. They become one.

Some time mind loses its consciousness and becomes identical with the object of meditation and meditator dissolves his personality in the sea of superpower, remains drowned and forgotten there till he becomes simply the instrument of superpower.

Someone not see or hear in state of Samadhi. There is no physical or mental consciousness only spiritual consciousness. There is only someone's true self and existence say superpower.

When the water dries up in a pool, the reflection of the sun in the water also vanishes. Similarly, when the mind melts in the superpower, the reflected consciousness or spirit or intelligence or sensation also vanishes

Someone experienced that there is infinite superpower bliss which is not a condition of inertia, forgetfulness or to destroy something completely so that nothing is left, but a state of absolute consciousness. Thus, it baffles all attempts at description. It is the final goal of all. It is liberation. It is self realization.

Someone experience immense silence and peace in every pore of one's being. One's whole being seems to have merged into superpower. It is not a state of sleep, because one is aware of everything. It also feels like a near-death state, because of one experience out-of-body experience. One can remain in that state from just a few minutes to days or more.

You should do meditation. The more you practice it, the deeper an experience it becomes. Finally, deep meditation will lead you to Samadhi, or oneness with superpower. You can start by fixing the mind for just 30-60 seconds on a particular object with focusing, or concentration and continue meditations becoming witness of your thoughts which ultimately take you to silence or peace of mind and Samadhi.

Someone experience a state where the mind loses its consciousness and identifies with the object of meditation and merge like a toy made of salt dissolves quickly in water, the mind is described as melting in the superpower in Samadhi.

You should start meditation without thinking. You try to be witness of thoughts and allow them to pass without any participation. Over a period you will become silent and thoughts will minimize and may not disturb you and ultimately you will experience state of Samadhi. Indian master said to practice more and more. You should be patience and continue.

You should keep in mind external worlds are created by lower mind and by controlling it the external world vanished. Person becomes on what try to meditating without affecting matter, space or time and reach to above all.

Prana Energy and Meditation

Silence and meditation increase prana energy flow to the body and help to reach up to Samadhi and keep healthy. It flows by 3, 20, 000 nadies in the whole body. If prana level in body increases disturbs the sleep but it is always good for spiritual and health. There are two types of energies in physical body called prana and mind or consciousness so every organ of the body there should be two channels supplying energy. It's found by modern physiology that two types of nervous systems are there, the sympathetic and the parasympathetic, and these two nervous systems are interconnected in each and every organ of the body. In the same way, every organ is supplied with the energy of prana and the energy of mind. The concept of prana is scientific but it is not breath or oxygen but original life force or internal energy.

The prana means constant motions which commence from mother's womb and maintain body's heat and life. There are three nadies in spinal cord called Ida, Pingala and Sushumna.Ida nadi represent the mental energy, Pingala prana energy and Sushumna spirit or spiritual awareness. These originate in mooladhara chakra situated at the perineum or cervix.

Remember Prana is not merely a philosophical concept; it is a physical substance and in the form of radioactive or electromagnetic waves exists even though we can't see them. It's observed that in the physical body, there are pranic waves and a pranic field. Everyone has a certain quantity of prana in their physical body and they utilize this in the course of their day to day activities throughout the life. When their prana level disturbed it cause sickness, and when they have plenty of prana, every part of the body maintain perfect health. If someone have an excess of prana, it can be transmitted to others for healing or magnetism or flow to ground some time which cannot be used and too excessive quantity.

The inner prana can be stimulated by the practice of pranayam or deep breathing and thereby increased to a greater quantity. The brain requires maximum prana for better functioning and to do meditation better way it needs plenty quantity. It is very essential to practice pranayam before commencing the meditation practice. Anulom vilom pranayam help to start Sushumna nadi which help to allow positive thoughts and improve meditation. If the supply of pranic fuel to the brain is not enough the mind becomes very restless and disturbed.

When the brain is not getting enough supply of prana, people suffer from nervous depression or nervous breakdown. The whole body perspires, there is trembling in every organ, one can't stand, their mind is unsteady and one is constantly thinking negative thoughts. One can't even sleep and don't like to talk or think. This state indicates that the brain is only receiving a very small quantity of prana and oxygen supply should be increased.

You should sit in steady asana for Anulom vilom pranayam. Close the right nostril with your finger or thumb and breath from the left nosetril, do as slow as possible till your lungs become full. You can release finger or thumb and close the left nostril and release it through right nosetril.You take breath from right nostril and release from left nosetril.This is called one Anulom vilom pranayam. You should try to do this practice 30-60 times before starting meditation.

Following picture shows how to seat and perform Anulom vilom pranayam.

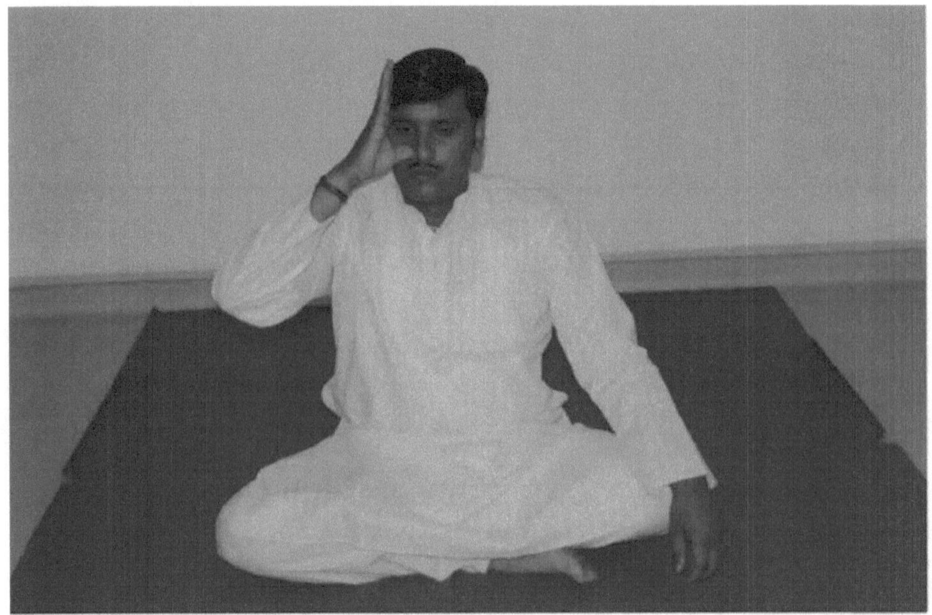

You should remember that not just by practicing a little pranayam can send a lot of prana to someone's brain. The process of supply and assimilation of prana into the brain is very complicated. The brain is a subtle instrument and it can only be enriched by the subtle form of prana and not the gross form and hence when you practice pranayam, you will have to convert the prana into a subtle force.

You should remember that deep breathing alone is not enough to stimulate prana. You can simulate your respiratory system and the blood circulation by breathing deeply but if you could examine the brain at that time, you would see that it is least affected. If you practice pranayam with concentration, as shown by scientific studies, the brainwaves undergo a significant change and the limbic system is also positively influenced.

Someone's brain can be split into two parts- the frontal brain and the posterior brain. The posterior brain is the instinctive brain which one has inherited through animal incarnations. The frontal brain is the seat of total consciousness. Someone breathe without awareness, the breath is registered in the posterior brain, but with awareness someone breath and consciously witnessing the whole process, then it registered by the conscious brain or the frontal brain.

The difference seems to be very simple, but its effect is very great. Most of the people breathe unconsciously like animals, children except who do practicing yoga. The pranic flow is being registered in the posterior brain as if in a computer. Once you become aware of your breath and you begin to conduct and control the breath in a particular fashion, immediately the frontal brain registers the influence. You should try to breathe with awareness to have better effect as described.

This fact has been revealed by scientific experiments and has led us to the following conclusion. Conscious breathing has an entirely different effect on the brain than unconscious breathing. Through unconscious breathing we are definitely able to feed the whole body with prana, but our brain is not getting enough prana for functioning and growth of it.

Someone cannot depend to avoid sicknesses of the brain and to develop the latent capacities of the brain or to initiate evolution of the brain on one's breathing old methods and follow and practice different forms of pranayam. Someone have to aware while breathing to come out such mental problems.

When you practice pranayam, the pranas are stimulated in the lower region of the body but you must have to force the pranic energy up. If you create a negative force which will push the pranic energy up through the spinal cord and pranayam should be practiced in coordination with specific bandhas to force pranic energy upward. The three bandhas which are incorporated into the practice of pranayam are jalandhara bandha, uddiyana bandha and moola bandha. They create a negative force like the ejecting force used to extract water from the well. When we practice pranayam with the bandhas ejecting force come in picture.

You can practice pranayam,generate prana in the lower region of the body and then push it up to the brain you must first practice moola bandha, then uddiyana bandha and finally jalandhara bandha. Moola bandha is contraction of the perineum, uddiyana bandha is contraction of the abdominal muscles and jalandhara bandha is the locking of the chin against the sternum. Prana compressed and pushed to the brain with the help of the subtle circulatory system.

As discussed earlier prana flows in 3, 20,000 nadis and are connected with chakras in spinal cord which are working as transformers or booster to push in the systems and allow flowing each and every organs of the body. If someone's body organ has short supply of prana become sick or malfunction body parts. This system is totally separate form blood circulation system.

Normally required quantity of prana is supplied to body organs to maintain good health. The importance of pranayam is to continuously generate a higher voltage of prana and sufficient quantity should be directed into the higher centers of the brain, via the above discussed nadies and pranic system. In this way, pranayam brings a higher reality to its experienced practitioner. It boosts the level of consciousness by activating and awakening the dormant centers and capacities of the left and right hemispheres of the evolving brain.

The other way to force and supply prana to the frontal portion of the brain is by the practice of Shambhavi mudra. Shambhavi mudra is centralizing the pupils of the eyes at the point between the two eyebrows. This practice is also known as mid-eyebrow centre gazing. When you practice Shambhavi mudra, the pranas are sucked up by force to force and supplied the frontal area of the brain. Indian master taught this method thounds of year ago.

You want to force sufficient prana in brain; you will have to practice pranayam very systematically. Pranayam is not just a matter of breathing in and breathing out in a particular way but Kumbhaka, retention of breath, is the actual cycle of pranayam. Inhalation and exhalation are just a normal process. In all the ancient yoga texts, Kumbhaka has been highly praised, and today scientists are acknowledging what the texts have claimed.

Retention of breath is done at two points when you have filled your lungs and secondly, when you empty your lungs called Retention(Antar Kumhaka) and Retention(Bahya Kumbhaka) which are important and they are so powerful that they can completely rejuvenate the whole brain.

In order to develop and provide sufficient quantity of prana shakti, certain practices have been formulated in many parts of the world and in India also. The Indian yogis have developed the science of prana which is called prana techniques. This is a very ancient and effective science which is still continued in India today.

Some people have more than required prana since birth time and they are able to transmit that prana out of the body to other people. You should keep in mind that all people may not have sufficient prana to cure sickness or heal. People can definitely awaken their own prana and give it to any part of the body that requires, wherever sickness occurs in the body or a deficiency of prana. If people can supply more prana to that part of the body they can heal and recover from the sickness. The process of healing is called self healing and if done to heal others is called spiritual healing.

Khumbaka pranayam discussed in earlier chapter so not repeated here so refer and practice to improve prana circulation and have better meditation, silence and peace of mind.

You can start distributing prana from ajna chakra to any part of the body you choose which is sick or required. If there is a problem with your fingers or your feet or any other part of the body, start sending prana there from ajna chakra. Either with the help of the breath or with the help of focusing your mind and try to push your prana to the affected part of the body and you will find that healing is taking place is called self healing. The principle of yoga and meditation is where is your mind pranic energy will flow and concentrate and perform healing. Chinese acupuncture or Japanese reiki are developed on this principle. I will discuss the same in later part.

Prana is not only the life force but it is also a very powerful healing force in the body that can even eradicate the most difficult physical problems. Moreover, the prana within us is the part of universal prana. I am not talking about positive and negative ions now; I am speaking of a metaphysical substance. This is called universal prana and your prana is same. If you can unite yourself with the universal prana, you can draw the required amount of prana whenever you need.

In order to tune yourself to this universal prana, you must be able to reach a higher state of meditation. When you control the breath, the mind is also controlled and the awareness becomes one-pointed. That one-pointed awareness is focused in the mid-eyebrow centre where the point is seen as a light. The light grows in intensity and becomes bigger and bigger until it completely envelops your consciousness. Then there is illumination all around you, and at this point you can connect yourself with the universal prana.

It is very difficult for us to tune ourselves to the universal prana because our awareness is very limited. Most of us only know about deep breathing, and we think that by breathing deeply fifty to a hundred times, we will get more and more Shakti. Of course we do, but we need a finer form of prana Shakti which can be used for awakening the brain.

Throughout your body there is a pranic field which is known as pranamaya kosha. You must know how to tune this pranamaya kosha with the universal prana. Your pranamaya kosha can be awakened by practicing pranayam correctly, by fasting or eating properly and by perfecting meditation on the mid-eyebrow centre. Then, when you are able to see that great enveloping light, you become the medium of the universal prana.

Thereafter, you can distribute this prana to those who are in short supply and it helps to purify your body also allowing more and more prana to yourself from universe.

Prana energy is name in Hindu. It's called "Chi" in Chinese and in Hebrew it's called "Ruash". This energy is vital force for life and increased in human body for getting peace and good quality of meditation and ultimately state of Samadhi.

It is also used for spiritual healing in many countries. It's called Reiki in Japan. Chinese it's called "Chi". China they invented acupuncture method in which normal electric power is step down to required by human body voltage and entered by fine pins to the body for healing or cure sickness.

I saw one girl of age about 10-12 years when I was attending one meditation program in India. She had a pinhole in inner part of internal wall of her heart. She was told for operation as final remedy. Somebody suggested her father to contact our spiritual healer. His father talked to our meditation practitioner for her daughter to give prana energy. Spiritual healer called her every day for 5-10 minutes for healing and continued for one month. She was advised to check her doctor after one month. She was found normal in medical checkup and came on stage while our meditation program with her medical report. Both were happy as operation was postponed and pinhole was cured.

Satypraksh Goyankaji had also migraine pain when he was in Burma. He learnt Vipassana meditation there and his migraine pain completely healed by 10 days meditation course. He has done great effort to spread Vipassana meditation all over the world later on.

Vishwamitra yogi in Rig-Veda described prana form is God or superpower which I like to put here. This is called Gayatri mantra in Indian spiritual practice.

That form of prana, which remove pains, joyful, best, glorious, which remove sin, Godlike form superpower we allow inner side and pry to divert our intelligence on correct path of life.

Some of yogi consider prana is a messenger of God but not God but every brain has different ideas so reader can decide and try to do meditation and experience silence and state of Samadhi.

Superpower is like an ocean of prana and true self or soul is a drop of it. People have inbuilt machinery called chakras to get enough prana from universe but that are not functioning properly. Everybody should do meditation to active chakras and get prana flow more and more. It will improve all the health related problems and also improve silence and meditation.

Internal energy comes out while meditation

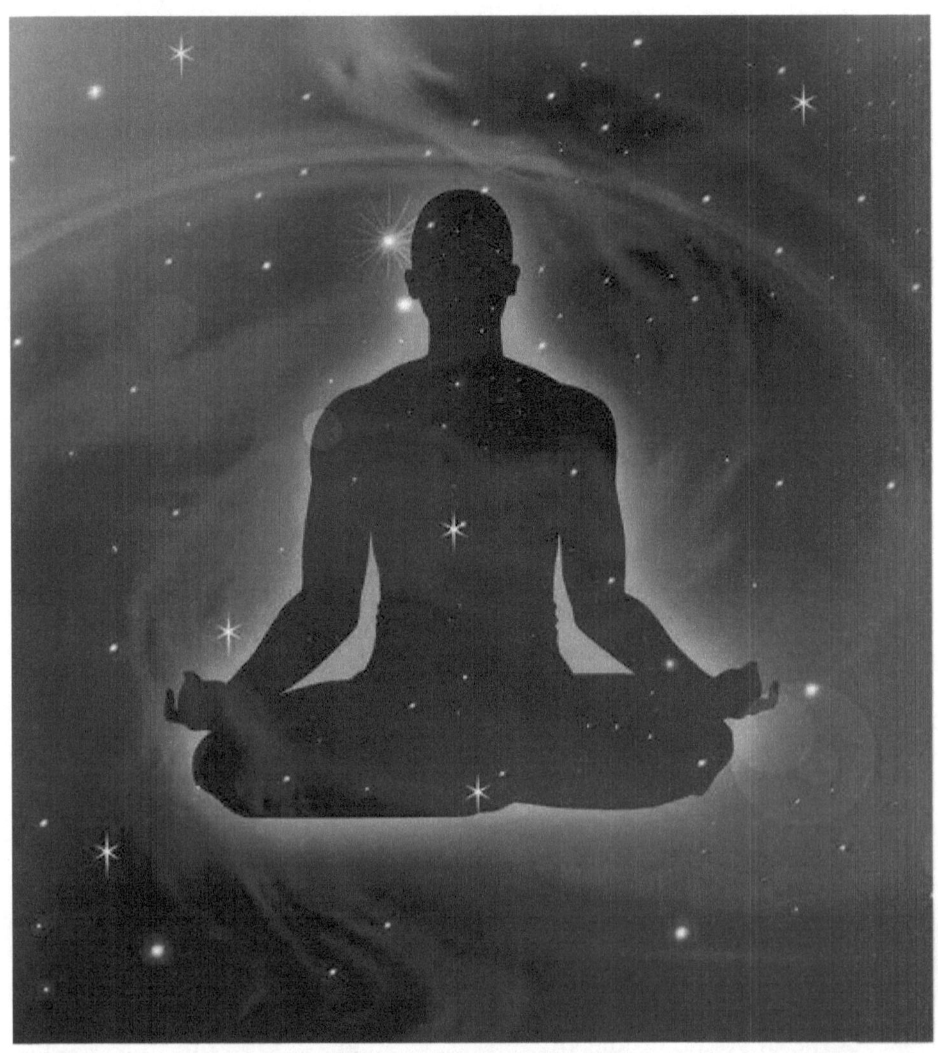

Energy flows to sick person from Spiritual healer.

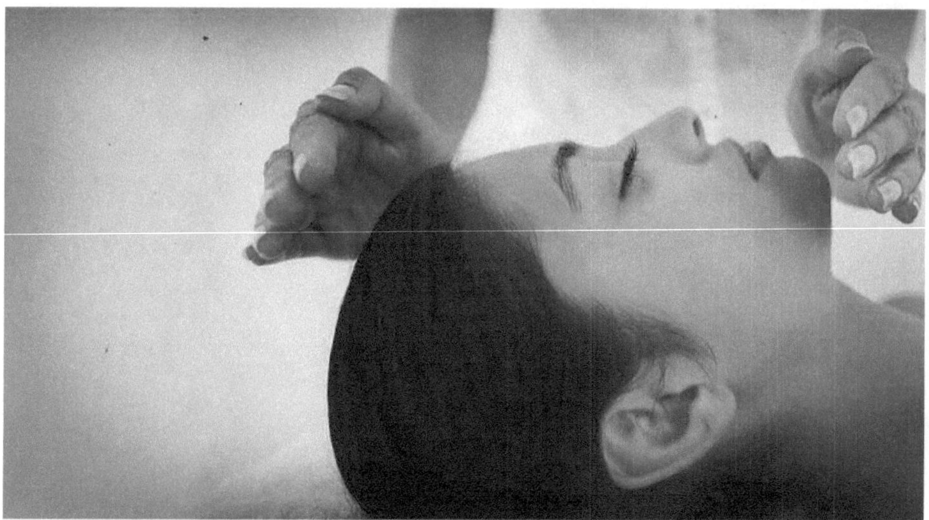